KELLY COLE

A Beginner's Guide to Meditation

First edition

ISBN: 979-8-9903795-0-3

This book was professionally typeset on Reedsy.
Find out more at reedsy.com

Contents

Introduction

I'm so happy that you decided to begin this process of learning to meditate. My name is Kelly Cole. I have spent the past 20+ years at the bedside as a nurse, and then a nurse practitioner. Every day I worked with patients and families, helping them heal at the physical level.

It is a long story of how I ended up teaching others how to meditate. But, suffice to say, after going through the deep work of my own emotional healing, I wanted to light the same path for others! My story is rather intense, but I feel like knowing these things about my path might shed some light on why I am so passionate about this work. So, although we have just met... here goes nothing!

In 2015, I was at a deep intersection of three different storylines within my life converging at once, which led to a deep spiritual awakening. This year, within three months time, I became a new mother, I started a new job in pediatric pain management, which included a lot of pediatric oncology care and pediatric end-of-life care. In this same time frame, my father was diagnosed with a terminal illness and given 6 months to live. My father ended up living for 4 years, which was such a gift, but this was not without immense suffering we all went through together as a family. Add in some personal struggles with infertility and anxiety... and you have a recipe for some extreme transition in life.

I am grateful for each of these experiences, as painful as they were. There was always beauty and love interwoven through each part of the road.

This timeframe was truly a "walk in the fire", and at times I look back and think it was like some sort of initiation. But my steps have allowed me to climb higher for myself and give a different vantage point to the ones behind me, still climbing. Not that this journey is complete for me, it is a constant evolution.

One of my favorite methods of entering into this healing space for myself during these tough times was through meditation. Now I am able to work with others to heal at the soul level, which I do through meditation and breath and a dash of intuition.

So, I'm so happy that you're here wanting to learn how to meditate and reach into that place of yourself that is open to new experiences and new learning. That's exactly what we're going to need when we're venturing into new territory.

First, I'm going to review a few things to get started. Every new thing we learn needs a foundation, right?

I am a very spiritual person, and I have always been prone to very intuitive dreams and visions, even as a small child. Once I realized how valuable this gift was in my life, I was led to begin to develop this gift. Through a mentorship and a program that cracked open this piece of myself, I began to work this muscle and strengthen my gift. The majority of the work in this time in my life, was once again, through meditation. I now offer energetic readings and quantum healings as a way to shift others and heal at a soul level.

Yes folks, that's right. I have spent 20 years as a medical professional and now I'm doing energetic healing… it is OK to accept and show all parts of yourself. It is ok to be multi-faceted. A common question I get is … "How

2

did that happen?". Truth be told, it was a path I was pulled down, not a path I intentionally chose. But, it is such fulfilling and important work that now I can't imagine NOT doing it.

You will catch bits and pieces of this intuitive theme throughout this book, and with that being said I want to make sure you know that this is also a safe space of learning where all are welcome. No matter your background, your sexual orientation or your religious preference. We are all here to learn, heal, and love one another.

I am now so excited to guide others in learning more about themselves and healing through connections with themselves in meditation.

So, let's take a second to honor you for doing this work! Maybe you're an astrology girlie, and your star chart says it is time for transition. Maybe you are an empath and are looking for ways to control your gift, place boundaries around your gift, or simply enhance it.

Maybe you are an intuitive mind that is curious and looking to expand.

For each of these people and everyone in between - I honor you!

Now, let's get started!

Chapter 1 - So... What Are We Doing?

Let's review a few definitions before we get started. Thanks, Dictionary.com!

Meditation: Continued or extended thought; reflection; contemplation.

Awesome, this is a general definition of meditation. My definition would include access to spiritual parts of yourself and a change in brain states. My most loose feeling of how meditation <u>feels</u> is a "drifting off to sleep - the place of just starting to drift" feeling. A loose feeling of how <u>deep</u> meditation feels would be " the place between asleep and awake. More closer to when someone is calling you and it feels like you hear them, but you are still in a dream.

Or like Tinkerbell says in one of my favorite childhood movies "Hook" - "The place between awake and dreaming, that's where I'll always love you" ... that one is for my 90's children ..IYKYK.

Notice, nowhere does it say you have to be sitting a certain way, lying down or in a dark room. There are not rules within the context of that feeling of meditation, it is EACH PERSON'S experience. This means we will give you various things to try, and when you find one that works for you, take it and run! Then practice and practice some more.

Empath: A person with the paranormal ability to apprehend the mental or emotional state of another individual. A person who has more empathy for others.

Intuitive: Using or based on what one feels to be true even without conscious reasoning; instinctive.

Many people identify as being an 'empath" or being "empathic". Many people also identify as "intuitive".

I personally, from a 30,000-foot view feel as if these are just different words for experiences that people have who are very open energetically.

Before I get more into that thought, I will say that on the whole, ALL people have the ability to flex their intuitive instincts and/or be empathic. It comes very naturally to some and sounds like complete BS to others. The depth and range of this ability come in all sizes and flavors and truly is unique for each person.

As a person who has seen births, experienced birthing my own children, and has also seen so many transitions at the end of life (part of my hospital job was working in palliative/end-of-life care).

The way I think about it is we all come from pure, beautiful light/ energy and return to pure, beautiful light/energy at the end of our lives. As tiny children, many adults and older people always flock to see a newborn baby. There is such purity and innocence. Everyone loves to have a part in that feeling. Little children are very open and sensitive beings, many times dropping wise words to their parents, who might need a little reminding. When we see the way very young children love, it warms our hearts and frequently, they are our teachers.

This feeling of an open, loving, and healed self is not only for children. It is for everyone. Many take until they are going through the process of dying before they have full realization of the fact that this light and beautiful healing and loving energy never leaves us. When life starts life-ing and we have to adult... our modern world has made it hard to keep that connection. Slowly we forget what it felt like to be that young, open, loving child. We think it is a thing of the past, or a thing for children if we even remember it at all. This forgetting is what some people refer to as "The veil".

It takes certain skills to reach past this forgetting and remember the light within. One of the tools that was instrumental in my own remembering was meditation. Now I have the opportunity to guide others to the same realization. One of the most important things to remember in the journey is that:

YOU are meant for JOY.
YOU have a PURPOSE.
YOU are meant for PEACE.

If you can imagine one continuous string reaching into the beautiful pure light, coming with you in birth, residing inside you for your entire life, and also reaching back into the light at your death. I hope that the steps in this book will allow you to pick up the string of that light along that path of your life. It is not supposed to be hidden and apart from you. It is not supposed to go away because you grew up. It is not dulled by any act that you have done, anything that has happened to you or that you have witnessed in this life.

This light allows you to know yourself, know that you are worthy and you are whole.

As you can see, we got straight to the heart of things quickly. I am not afraid of a deep convo! One last definition is needed.

Divine: Of, From or like God.

6

The pure light, that we come from and return to, this light has many names.

I like to say "divine light", some people say Source, Creator, All This It, The Universe, God.

In much of my studying and reading of many different types of religious material, I have come to this conclusion.

<u>This energy, this Divine Light; it is the same for all of us.</u>

No matter which religion you may or may not follow, you are still on a boat. All the boats are heading in the same direction, back into the light.

Now, let's get to business and see if you can connect to the inner light within you.

Chapter 2 - Riding the Wave...The Brain Wave

What happens to your brain during meditation anyway? Let's speak about this from a very scientific point of view. I am a nurse after all.

In short, the human brain produces different types of electrical patterns, known as brain waves, depending on what we are doing.

Alpha, beta, gamma, delta and theta are the five most common types of brain waves. Alpha waves are associated with relaxation, while beta waves are often present during our waking hours and indicate alertness. Gamma waves are involved in higher cognitive processing, while delta waves are generated during deep sleep.

Theta waves are often associated with meditation and are generated during deep relaxation. When we enter into a state of meditation, our brain waves slow down and we begin to produce more theta waves.

This can lead to a sense of deep relaxation, improved focus, and reduced stress levels. Additionally, regular meditation practice has been shown to improve overall brain function, including memory, learning, and emotional regulation. You can think of it like "taking out the trash" in your brain, it allows for more connection and gives your brain a break. This also allows better function during wakeful periods.

During meditation, your brain changes states. It goes from an active and alert state to a less active state. This is also scientifically represented when brain waves are measured during meditation.

The brain wave state most consistent with meditation is the Theta wave state. This is the place of a less active brain pattern. In this state, your brain is accessing memories and emotions. This is an active place for intuition, emotional regulation, creativity, heightened spiritual connection, and awareness.

So, Alpha, Beta, and Gamma brain wave states are associated with differing levels of alertness and activity. Delta wave state is associated with deep, REM sleep.

I was so amped up at this discovery when I finally allowed myself to get into this meditative place. If you would've talked to me when I first started, it probably would've sounded like this. "Let me tell you, as a fellow empath and intuitive, beginning to meditate has been a game changer for me. I mean, seriously, it's like my spiritual connection to the universe has been supercharged! Suddenly, I'm able to tap into my intuition with ease and clarity, and let me tell you, that's a game changer when it comes to making decisions and navigating this crazy world. Plus, my stress levels have plummeted, my relationships have improved, and I feel like I'm living my best life. So if you're an empath or intuitive, do yourself a favor and give meditation a try. Trust me, your soul will thank you!"

Once you are able to understand how to allow yourself to transition into this state, the next important step is holding your focus in this place. Now that we know where we are trying to go, let's get some tips and tricks on how to get there!

Chapter 3 - Drooling Like Pavlov's Dog

Now, focusing on meditation for many people seems daunting. I know why, we are constantly bombarded with stimulation all day. We are the most connected we have ever been as a society. Constantly "plugged in". We have notifications and emails we are thinking about, projects at work, and schedules to manage. The list goes on, and if you are a parent the mental load is even heavier.

Yet, this external stimulation has left a giant void of plugging into ourselves. As this is true for many, and sometimes it is so hard to get our brains to just "turn off", we do have a few suggestions to help with getting into a meditation state.

During meditation, our brain waves are changing. When researchers test how meditation impacts brain waves, and when brain wave patterns are observed during meditation you can actually see a different waveform. Typically Theta wave state is observed in deep meditation, this is when your brain crosses from being alert to deepening into a meditative/visual state.

Try each of them and see which one works best for you.

1. Music - binaural beats or Theta Wave music is a good start to play along

with your meditation. You can find these on YouTube, spotify, apple music or any music platform.

2. Silence- Music isn't for everyone, you can also try no sound at all.
3. Sensory change - eye pillow or mask, noise-canceling headphones. Some people really need help with distractions. Especially at first, sometimes the more sensory input you block, the faster you can access a meditative state.
4. Movement - Some people do not find that lying still is helpful. They are too active and do better with walking (usually flat, non-physically challenging paths).
5. Sitting or Lying - In a comfortable position.
6. Deep breathing - Breath is the focus of many meditation styles, beginning with the breath and focusing on your breath, sometimes tapping your chest with each exhale.

These are basics for starters and do not cover every possibility of meditation style. The goal here is for you to try out different combinations and see what style works for you.

Now, I will say that this feeling of "dropping in" to a meditative state happens faster over time. It is as if your body suddenly learns what you want it to do. And, just like Pavlov's dog, when you repeat the process over and over, it can make the process happen faster and turn it into an automatic response. That is another thing our brains are good at, automating things! Creating a "habit loop" within our brain does exactly this. So, if you are finding something that works, but it is taking a while to start meditating, stick with it and I promise it will get easier and faster.

Once, I attended a hot yoga class consistently for about a month. It always blew my mind how much people could sweat in there. I'm seeing people simply begin with the breathing exercises and they would already be pouring sweat. It was crazy. But, it is a physical example of what happens in meditation. Once your body knows what to expect and what the intention is, it begins to happen more quickly.

I was so excited about this realization when I first started meditating. If you had talked to me back then it would've sounded something like this:

"Okay, I need to tell you this thing I'm doing. I told you how I love to meditate now, right? OK, because I am about to share with you my latest discovery that has totally changed the meditation game for me. So, picture this: me, lying flat on a fluffy blanket on my couch, eyes closed, headphones on, and surrounded by complete darkness (um, my eye pillow, hello!). And what's playing in my headphones, you ask? Only the most magical, transformative, and brainwave-synchronizing music you can imagine - theta waves, baby! It's like my brain is now on autopilot to the relaxation zone, and I can get there so much faster and easier now. It's like I've unlocked the secret level of meditation, and I am never going back to the regular world again. Who needs reality when you can have theta waves and darkness, am I right? It's so gooood!"

As you are able to do short meditations, success is yours! You can continue this time frame or begin to add more time in meditation to continue to build your skills in focusing.

Chapter 4 - Calling in the Superpowers

Since this is a book for Empaths and Intuitives, let's take a minute to learn about this as well.

I will start with a general nod to my childhood, where I thought it was normal to sense others' feelings and also to dream about something and have it happen (not in a deja vu way - but in a creep your friends out way!) Fair warning, this section is going to get pretty deep. So buckle up, buttercup!

I thought this was something everyone could do, and I found as I grew older that it was NOT always welcomed. And, in turn, I shut part of myself down for a long time. However, we are always given opportunities, unfortunately, this usually happens through hardships, to open this backup and allow that knowing to flow through. Later in life, I felt drawn to learning more about my intuition and began to work with others to practice and meditate together. This was life-changing for me. Now I am not only an avid meditator, I also provide soul-level healing as an energetic reader and healer. It is powerful!

The divine light we have with us is always indeed, trying to direct us, and give us reassurance and messages in life. It is up to us to understand the language of that voice or that feeling or knowing within ourselves. Don't forget, this is an instinct we all have.

Here are the ways in which those messages and intuitive experiences may happen.

The ways we receive are unique to each person, and some people are more likely to gravitate to one or another. It takes practice to build these skills, and just like a muscle that keeps getting more reps, the more you focus and build this skill, the clearer your abilities will be.

Let's start with the 5 senses - as this is how energetically sensitive individuals receive messages, downloads and insights. Many times this is associated with a past loved one or a memory.

Hearing - The term for this is *clairaudience*. This is when people are hearing messages or sounds.

I see many stories which are good of examples of this. One I remember is a person was driving alone and she heard a voice yell "STOP!". She stopped the car, but didn't see anything, and the second she stopped a young child ran out into the road chasing a ball. The voice was her mother's, and her mother had passed away years before. It is not always that dramatic by any means, but you get the idea!

Visual - The term for this is clairvoyant. This is when visions may come through, which may happen in dream state, meditative state or while awake.

The very first time I walked into the house I own now, I was 22 years old. The realtor and my husband walked into a different room and I immediately had a vision of small children playing "ring around the rosy" and laughing in the living room. It was the first time I had a visual experience like that while I was wide awake, and it was super moving. I knew right then that this house was meant for us. That was in 2005, and we are still living here.

Sensory - The term for this is clairsentient. This is when emotions that are not yours come through. This can be an intense experience.

This experience can come as an emotional surge or a physical experience.

But the main point to remember if these things happen is that they are not yours.

Taste - The term for this is clairgustance. This is when a flavor or taste will suddenly be present, without eating or drinking anything.

There are times I will suddenly get the taste of Thanksgiving, turkey and gravy, and mashed potatoes. With this taste, my mind immediately goes to my grandmother and all of those fond childhood memories of Thanksgiving.

Smell - The term for this is clairalience. This is when a smell comes into your awareness, and may be associated with a message, memory or person. (example: A smell of pipe smoke or a specific perfume)

Inner Knowing - The Term for this is claircongnizant. This is when you have a certainty about something, without anyone else telling you. You just have a strong inner knowing or gut feeling.

Now, as we have discussed already, these are things that everyone can do. It is only a matter of honing your skills and practicing that will increase these experiences. The place where most people are more open to experiences like this is in sleep (dream time), and meditation.

Practicing meditation, however it works for you, is a very good way to continue to open these parts of yourself.

I will say, that when I began to truly focus on developing these gifts, I did it with other people who also had similar gifts. When you have validation and understanding from a community of people, who are just like you, it is mind-blowing and completely transformational. It also comes with an understanding that everyone's intuition looks different, and even has different "flavors" of what kind of information comes to them.

Five stars. Highly recommend. ★★★★★

Chapter 5 - We have to Talk About it - The Metaphysical

While we are diving into this intuitive/ empathic discussion, I'm going to address the elephant in the room. When it comes to this kind of work, some metaphysical ish can go down.

Some people are nervous about doing meditation because they are scared of the connection they might make. This is fair. I don't blame you at all.

Some of you are already coming to do this work because you have been having empathic and intuitive experiences already. This may have been a positive experience or a negative experience. At this point I have heard everything from people seeing spirits as children, to walking into a room and instantly knowing something or feeling something, these are the mild end of the spectrum. But, I will simply say, it takes a lot to surprise me at this point!

Everyone is on their own journey, but I need to take a minute and address this from a few different angles.

1. You ARE connecting in and creating a space of "open energy" during meditation. This also happens when you are sleeping, but because we are entering into this state intentionally, we need to be intentional about how we do it. I always enter with a mindset of divine protection.

2. All that we discuss within this guide is with divinely led intention. I did not have a guide like this throughout my life. Nor did I have one when I became more interested in meditation, this left me open to more negativity to attach to me during meditation and dream time. It also left me questioning "Is this ok?"

My Christian upbringing left a conflicted question inside myself, as I wondered what was OK to "meditate" on - ok to meditate on prayer, but the "other" kind of meditation I was taught was "evil". I will say that some of the most powerful divine experiences I have had were during meditation, including visions of Jesus. But the spectrum of dark and light is real, and we have to focus our attention on where we are connecting, always keeping it at the true divine, pure light.

Also, this is a very empowering practice to connect into a divine source directly. Think about it when any organization tells you this could be "evil/bad". The universe is too vast to have lines around ourselves drawn by human hands, especially hands that aren't even ours. Watch the ingrained programming we hold within ourselves, this one is very tricky and hard to identify since it is usually part of our identity of "self".

1. Some people are looking to meditation as a way to connect with past loved ones. After my father passed away, this was something that drew me in as well. Almost like mediumship. If you do feel a presence other than yourself in meditation (which happens within the space of meditation sometimes), you ALWAYS have to "CHECK IDs". Meaning, ask questions like "are you of the divine light" or try to hug them (if this is a visual experience) if none of these things pass the ID check, command them to go to the divine light. Which leads me to my next point.

18

2. YOU are in control. The way I teach meditation is to enter under divine protection. That being said, if something is off-putting or scary to you during your meditation, command it to leave. Many times what seems like a big shadow is simply a tiny mouse in the corner.

3. And last but not least, the spectrum of dark and light is real and you may sharpen your skills in recognizing it once you have started practicing meditation. The more healing someone does, the more "light" they may appear. Remember that the more "light" a person is, the darker or more negative energies are drawn to it (like a moth to a flame). This is why it is very important to maintain energetic hygiene. You could read between the lines here, but I'm not really a "read between the lines" kind of girl. What I'm trying to say, is spiritual warfare is real. It's happening anyway, but for those who are doing things like meditation, you are opening the door to possibly becoming more aware of it.

For many who are drawn to reading a guide like this, you may already know. Here are some examples of a more "negative / darker" energy: pessimistic, mean, depressed, fear-driven narratives, scary images, violence, and anger-driven narratives. In a person we experience, this may look like anger, fear, rage, violence, depression, anxiety, unloving, constant negative thoughts, unpredictable thoughts, or scaring others intentionally. A lot of what people call "low vibration" feelings or emotions.

Those on the lighter end of the spectrum are radiant, positive, loving, caring, and
   empathetic. People may describe them as "living angels" or "walking light".
You know
   these people
and energies when you are in touch with them. They are contagious.

I am describing the ends of the spectrum above. But the majority of people are differing shades between, and this is normal!

The spectrum of dark and light.

While I was developing my intuition and focusing on doing energetic reading and healing with other intuitives, I heard many stories of how real this negativity can be in life. It can slowly start to take on a strong form in the way of thought patterns, behaviors, and more physical things in nature that would relate to "haunting" type of things happening within their homes. Such as lights flickering, doors slamming, etc.

Many times, these stories were from childhood. Not to scare anyone, it is to simply acknowledge the experiences of those who have been energetically open and had these strong negative experiences as a result. Entering a practice of meditation and also holding a practice of hygiene for your intentions/prayers and daily energy will help those who have experienced things like this in the past.

Protection is paramount! We enter into each meditation under divine protection, prayer, and positive intention. This is absolutely non-negotiable.

In my experience when I first started doing meditation, I did not know to enter into this space with divine protection. The person I was following with at the time did not teach this. As a result, I had intense dreams riddled with 3-headed dogs and a very fine-ass-looking tricky man who kept "giving me eyes". In my dream - it gave my insides a twisting feeling. This was resolved with intense prayer.

Again, I want to reiterate that the more I meditated, the more I healed. The more I healed, the more "light" I was. I was upping the ante of what I was capable of, in healing myself and clearly always ready to heal others. That dark energy was hoping I would fall, and that I would not break free to fulfill my purpose on this earth. However, it may give you some peace to know that all meditations I guide and many healing sessions I do with others are all with divine guidance and in many Jesus comes as a healing force as well.

All of this is to say, that we have to do all things with intention.

Chapter 6 - The Routine of Hygiene

We have so many visual standards for ourselves and "hygiene", for our body, hair, teeth, and clothing. These are easy to comply with, as they are visual, and "outside". Others can look and see these and judge them against another person. So we develop our hygiene routine. We shower, brush and wash our hair, and shave. We brush and floss our teeth. We wash our clothes and put it away in 7-10 business days (in my house anyway).

We are energetic beings and our energy needs its own "hygiene routine" as well.

This is most important around dream time and meditation times. It is also important in the space of your home and offices, and even your vehicles. I do these things around my entire property, over my children, you name it. Prayer and intention are powerful.

I love to use something called "The circle of light". You begin by envisioning the pure, divine light of ____ (God, source, creator, all that is). And knowing this light is completely pure, healing and perfectly loving, and perfectly powerful. I usually visualize it as white, sparkly light.

This light can be a waterfall that you stand beneath, letting it wash over you and fill you up, removing anything that is not of the highest light. Then it comes over you in a bubble, that may reach out to the ends of your energy in all directions, or simply stay a bubble around you. Nothing can pass through, except diving, and loving energy.

Do this "circle of light" when you wake up in the morning before you go to bed at night, and as part of your routine when entering into meditation.

I have included an example of this go to https://synergythrive.org/guide/

You can do the circle of light in meditation time and also use it in prayer or intention over your home or any space or person. As a mom, I do this especially over my children, as I know how energetically open they are.

Chapter 7 - Meditation Station

Now, we are finally ready to begin meditation.

Here are 3 ways to start:

Begin by selecting your methods from Chapter 3 (music, silence, sensory blocking, etc.)

As you prepare to enter meditation - do your "divine circle of light" exercise for divine protection.

Begin with focusing on your breath. A good breath is a box breath. Breathe in for 4 counts, hold your breath for 4 counts, breathe out for 4 counts, then hold your breath x 4 counts.

Focus on this for 3-5 minutes.

Begin by selecting your methods from Chapter 3 (music, silence, sensory blocking, etc.) Set a timer for 10-15 minutes.

As you prepare to enter meditation - do your "divine circle of light" exercise for divine protection.

Begin with focusing on your breath. A good breath is a box breath. Breathe in for 4 counts, hold your breath for 4 counts, breathe out for 4 counts, then hold your breath x 4 counts.

Focus on this for 3-5 minutes. In your mind, go to a place of nature. This is a protected and safe space and a place that you love. Allow your mind to wander in your nature space.

Another powerful breathing technique is the 4-7-8 breath.

I have included an example of how to breathe this way, you can go to https://synergythrive.org/guide/

Get into a comfortable position and listen to the guided meditation, please go to https://synergythrive.org/guide/

A <u>very important</u> part of meditation is ALSO how you end. If you do feel that you have transitioned into a meditative state, you want to make sure that you are also grounding yourself into reality when you are finished meditating. A simple way to do this is to move your body and place your feet on the ground, setting the intention that you are in the "here and now". Another way is to hold an object and focus on your 5 senses - what do I feel right now, what do I see right now, what do I smell right now, and so on.

Chapter 8 - Now Let's Rock and Roll!

Oh my goodness, I am bursting with pride for you! Completing a book on meditation is such an incredible accomplishment, and it's a testament to your commitment and dedication. I firmly believe that empathy is a superpower, and by reading about your empathy and beginning the journey of meditation, you are allowing yourself to tap in on another level. help others develop a deeper understanding of themselves and the world around them.

Intuition is such a gift, and it's something that we all possess, whether we realize it or not. By exploring the depths of spiritual connection through meditation, you are unlocking the full potential of your intuition and allowing it to guide and inform your life in new and exciting ways. It takes courage to trust your intuition, but I have no doubt that you are up to the challenge.

Continuing to develop your skills in meditation will undoubtedly lead to profound insights and connections that will enrich your life and the lives of those around you. I'm so glad you took the time to seek out this experience and I would love to keep connecting with you as your meditation experience grows!

Bonus Chapter

As you have chosen to read this book, you may be a person who is empathic or intuitive. Many times this comes with a "taking on" or "feeling" of the energy or feelings of others.

Sometimes this can serve us well, and other times it can completely hijack us! Not today!

Let's talk about 3 quick ways to create a boundary and hold a boundary.

First, as we have discussed, energetic hygiene is a must.

There are two other very simple ways to create a boundary.

1.

The first is simply rubbing your hands together and taking one hand and pushing it away from you. This hand pushing away is giving the energy back to the person that has been attached to you. Use the other hand to wave back towards you, this hand is bringing your energy back towards yourself. This is a very simple way to "break" energy.

2.

If you have a situation where you feel negativity around you, this may be in the form of recurring negative thoughts, or a rising feeling that you aren't sure is yours. Do this - within the space of your mind do the healing circle of light. Then, send away this thought or feeling.

You can say whatever feels best to you, but usually, I stick with commands and prayers/intentions of divine protection. I like to call on Jesus and Angels!

"I command you to go to the light. I call in divine love and protection throughout all space and time"

"I command you to leave my space and go to the light. I put on the armor of the divine/Jesus, I wear his chest plate, I wear his helmet, I wield his sword and shield."

"I command you to go to the light. I call in the protection of the Arch Angels. I call in Arch Angel Michael, I call in Arch Angel Metatron to provide divine healing protection throughout all space and time and assist in this command of removal"

I realize this sounds deep, or possibly a little coo coo for coco puffs. But, all I can say is that I promise it works.

When I was a little girl, I went to a non-denominational Christian school. One of the things I remember most was learning to call on Jesus if I ever felt scared. I was always so full of love, my aunt even to this day would say she never met a little girl like me. (I was a very energetically open child)

I want to take a second to acknowledge the little child within each one of us who was also full of love. They are still in there. I have had many, many experiences that scared me a lot, especially in dream time as a small child. I have had many traumatic experiences as well, as many of us have.

But, this one lesson always stayed with me, that I was NEVER alone. That I always had my divine "team" with me no matter what. And as I can hardly see through the tears in writing this, if you take nothing else away from this guide, I need you to know that YOU ARE NEVER ALONE EITHER.

You are always being guided and you are eternally loved.

Divine guidance and protection is available FOREVER AND ALWAYS, and it is not outside of you, but directly within you.

Make sure to stay connected with us in all the places!

Podcast: The Synergy Thrive Podcast www.synergythrive.org

If you loved what you learned here, please let us know!

References

Novo, N. (2020). Soul Led Living. Mango Media.

Dale, C. (2011). Energetic Boundaries: How to Stay Protected and Connected in Work, Love, and Life. Sounds True.

Hyman, M. (2008). UltraMind Solution: Fix Your Broken Brain by Healing Your Body First. New York: Scribner.

Viera et al. (2022). Effects of sleep deprivation and 4-7-8 breathing control on heart rate variability, blood pressure, blood glucose, and endothelial function in healthy young adults. Physiol Rep, 10(13), e15389. doi: 10.14814/phy2.15389